COMPLETE GUIDE TO UNDERSTANDING ARTHROSCOPY

Mastering Keyhole, Essential Insight To Techniques, Procedures, And Innovations In Minimally Invasive Surgery

KLEIN HOYLE

© [KLEIN HOYLE] [2024]

All rights reserved.

No part of this book may be reproduced, distributed, or transmitted in any form or by any means, including photocopying, recording, or other electronic or mechanical methods, without the publisher's prior written permission, with the exception of brief quotations in critical reviews and certain other noncommercial uses permitted by copyright law.

Disclaimer

The content in this book is based on the author's expertise and comprehension of the topic. The author has no affiliation or link with any corporation, business, or person. This book is meant to give general information and educational material only, and it should not be interpreted as professional medical advice. Always seek the advice of a skilled healthcare expert if you have any queries about medical issues or treatments. The author and publisher expressly disclaim any responsibility resulting directly or indirectly from the use or use of the information included in this book.

Table of Contents

CHAPTER 1 11
- Introduction To Arthroscopy 11
- What Is Arthroscopy? 11
- History And Development Of Arthroscopic Surgery 11
- Benefits Of Arthroscopy 12
- Common Conditions Treated With Arthroscopy 13
  - 1. Meniscal tears: 14
  - 2. Rotator Cuff Tears: 14
  - 3. ACL Reconstruction: 14
  - 4. Cartilage Damage: 15

CHAPTER 2 17
- Anatomy Basics 17
- Understanding Joint Anatomy 17
- The Function Of Ligaments, Tendons, And Cartilage 19
- How Joints Function 20
- Importance Of Joint Health 22

CHAPTER 3 25
- Preparing For Arthroscopic Surgery 25

Preoperative Exams And Testing 25
Medications And Diet Restrictions 27
Arranging Transportation And Assistance 28
Mental Preparation For Surgery 29

CHAPTER 4 33
Arthroscopic Procedure 33
Overview Of The Surgical Process 33
Anesthesia Options 34
Insertion Of Arthroscopes And Instruments 35
Visualizing And Treating Joints 36

CHAPTER 5 39
Recovery And Rehabilitation 39
Immediate Post-Operative Care 39
Pain Management Strategies 40
Physical Therapy Exercises 41
Gradual Return To Normal Activities 43

CHAPTER 6 45
Complications And Risks 45
Potential Complications Of Arthroscopy 45
Infection Prevention Measures 47
Managing Postoperative Pain And Discomfort .. 49

Signs Of Complications To Watch For 51

CHAPTER 7..55

Arthroscopy Of Specific Joints 55

Knee Arthroscopy: Procedures And Results 55

Shoulder Arthroscopy: Indications And Benefits 58

Hip Arthroscopy: Applications And Limitations. 60

Ankle And Wrist Arthroscopy: Special Considerations 63

CHAPTER 8..65

Advanced Techniques And Innovation 65

Emerging Technology In Arthroscopic Surgery ..65

Minimally Invasive Approaches.....................66

Future Trends In The Field 67

CHAPTER 9..71

Lifestyles And Prevention 71

Maintaining Joint Health With Exercise And Diet 71

Injury Prevention Strategies.........................72

Ergonomics And Joint-Friendly Habits............74

The Need For Regular Check-Ups And Screenings 75

CHAPTER 10 77
   After Surgery: Long-Term Joint Care 77
   Follow-Up Appointments, Monitoring 77
   Managing Chronic Conditions 78
   Coping With Limitations And Adaptive Activities 79
   Resources And Support For Maintaining Joint Health 80
   Conclusion 82
THE END 85

ABOUT THIS BOOK

The "Complete Guide to Understanding Arthroscopy" is a thorough compendium that delves into the complexities of arthroscopic surgery in great depth and clarity. As readers begin their trip via this educational tome, they are welcomed with an illuminating investigation in Chapter 1, which explains the essential ideas underpinning arthroscopy. From tracing its historical beginnings to describing its many advantages, this chapter provides a solid basis for understanding the importance of this surgical method in contemporary medicine.

Moving beyond theoretical foundations, Chapter 2 explains the fundamental anatomy behind arthroscopic operations. Through a detailed examination of joint components and their critical functions, readers get a great understanding of the complex interaction of ligaments, tendons, and cartilage, recognizing the need to maintain joint health. This anatomical introduction flows effortlessly into Chapter 3, where the precise preparations required for arthroscopic surgery are methodically described. From pre-operative examinations to mental preparedness, this chapter acts as a compass, leading patients and practitioners through the preoperative maze.

As readers go into the core of arthroscopy—the surgical realm—Chapter 4 provides a panoramic view of the procedure. The delicate dance of anesthetic, equipment, and imaging is shown here, demystifying the surgical ballet for those unfamiliar with it. The next chapters provide a tapestry of healing (Chapter 5), risk reduction (Chapter 6), joint-specific subtleties (Chapter 7), technology frontiers (Chapter 8), lifestyle treatments (Chapter 9), and long-term joint stewardship (Chapter 10).

Notably, this epic work distinguishes out not just for its encyclopedic scope, but also for its embrace of cutting-edge advances and caring guidance. From developing technology to holistic lifestyle recommendations, each chapter acts as a lighthouse, exposing routes to better patient outcomes and long-term joint health. Whether navigating the maze of rehabilitation or considering the possibilities of long-term joint care, readers are encouraged by a wealth of information and practical advice.

In essence, the "Complete Guide to Understanding Arthroscopy" goes beyond the scope of a typical guidebook; it emerges as a valued confidant, a steady partner on the difficult journey toward joint health and repair. This groundbreaking text, with its academic explanation and caring attitude, not only provides readers with the necessary information but also instills them with the strength and optimism required to navigate the surgical adventure with confidence and fortitude.

CHAPTER 1

Introduction To Arthroscopy

What Is Arthroscopy?

Arthroscopy is a minimally invasive surgical treatment for diagnosing and treating joint disorders. It entails putting a tiny camera called an arthroscope into the joint via a small incision. This enables the surgeon to see inside the joint on a screen and execute a variety of surgical operations using specialist devices.

History And Development Of Arthroscopic Surgery

The earliest efforts to view the interior of joints with basic devices occurred in the early twentieth century, marking the beginning of arthroscopic surgery. However, it wasn't until the 1960s and 1970s that arthroscopy methods and tools improved significantly, allowing for more accurate and successful surgeries.

Dr. Masaki Watanabe is credited with creating the modern arthroscope in the 1970s, which transformed the field of orthopedic surgery.

Since then, arthroscopic surgery has evolved with advancements in imaging technology, instruments, and surgical procedures. Today, it is often utilized in orthopedic medicine to diagnose and treat a variety of joint disorders.

Benefits Of Arthroscopy

One of the key advantages of arthroscopic surgery is its limited invasiveness. Compared to conventional open surgery, arthroscopy uses smaller incisions, which results in less tissue damage, less discomfort, and quicker recovery periods for patients. Furthermore, since the surgeon can see the joint directly, arthroscopy enables more exact diagnosis and treatment of joint disorders.

Another benefit of arthroscopy is its adaptability. It is effective for treating a variety of joint disorders, including ligament and tendon injuries, cartilage damage, arthritis, and loose bodies inside the joint. In many circumstances, arthroscopic surgery may successfully treat these concerns while requiring less risk and delay than standard open surgery.

Furthermore, arthroscopy is often done as an outpatient procedure, allowing patients to return home the same day as their operation. This eliminates the need for hospitalization and cuts healthcare expenses.

Common Conditions Treated With Arthroscopy

Arthroscopy is often used to treat disorders involving the knee, shoulder, hip, ankle, elbow, and wrist joints. Some of the most frequent problems addressed with arthroscopic surgery are:

1. **Meniscal tears:** Tears in the cartilage of the knee joint, known as menisci, are a common cause of knee discomfort and instability. Arthroscopic surgery may be done to trim or repair a torn meniscus, which relieves symptoms and restores knee function.

2. **Rotator Cuff Tears:** Tears in the shoulder tendons, especially the rotator cuff, may cause discomfort, weakness, and a restricted range of motion. Arthroscopic procedures enable accurate repair of rotator cuff injuries, frequently resulting in enhanced shoulder function and less discomfort.

3. **ACL Reconstruction:** ACL injuries are prevalent, particularly among sports. Arthroscopic ACL restoration includes replacing the damaged ligament with a graft, which is often taken from the patient's own body or a donor. This surgery helps to stabilize the knee and restore normal function.

4. Cartilage Damage: Damage to the articular cartilage that covers the ends of the bones in a joint may cause discomfort, swelling, and reduced movement. Arthroscopic procedures, such as microfracture or cartilage transplantation, may be utilized to repair or replace damaged cartilage, which promotes healing and alleviates symptoms.

5. Synovitis is inflammation of the synovial lining of a joint that causes pain, swelling, and stiffness. Arthroscopic synovectomy is the removal of inflammatory synovial tissue, which relieves symptoms and prevents additional joint injury.

6. Loose bodies are particles of bone or cartilage inside a joint that may cause discomfort, locking, and catching sensations. Arthroscopic surgery may remove these loose bodies, restoring normal joint function and relieving discomfort.

Overall, arthroscopic surgery provides various advantages for patients with joint disorders, such as less intrusive treatments, shorter recovery periods, and better results. Arthroscopy restores joint function and relieves pain by treating common disorders such as meniscal tears, rotator cuff tears, ACL injuries, cartilage loss, synovitis, and loose bodies, enabling patients to resume normal activities with minimum downtime.

CHAPTER 2

Anatomy Basics

Understanding Joint Anatomy

Understanding joint anatomy is essential in arthroscopy. Joints are the sites where two or more bones come together, providing mobility and flexibility. They are classified into many varieties, including hinge joints (like the knee), ball-and-socket joints (like the hip), and pivot joints (like the neck). Each joint type enables distinct motions required for everyday tasks.

Let us now go further into the components of a joint. Cartilage is a smooth, slippery tissue found at the ends of bones in a joint. Cartilage works as a cushion, minimizing friction between bones during movement and absorbing stress. Ligaments surround the joint and are thick, fibrous bands that link bones, giving stability and restraining excessive movement.

Tendons, on the other hand, link muscles and bones, allowing the muscles to move the bones around the joint.

When all of these components work together properly, the joint runs smoothly, allowing for a broad range of motion without pain or discomfort. However, when any portion of the joint is damaged, whether via accident, illness, or wear and tear, it may cause pain, stiffness, and decreased mobility.

Understanding joint anatomy is the cornerstone for arthroscopic operations. Orthopedic surgeons may effectively diagnose and treat a variety of joint disorders utilizing minimally invasive procedures if they understand how each component interacts inside the joint.

The Function Of Ligaments, Tendons, And Cartilage

Ligaments, tendons, and cartilage all play important roles in joint function and stability. Ligaments act like the body's natural cords, keeping bones together and limiting excessive movement. They give stability and support, allowing for regulated motions inside the joint and preventing it from injury.

Tendons, on the other hand, act as connections between muscles and bones. When muscles contract, tendons transfer the force to the bones, creating movement at the joint. Without tendons, even the strongest muscles would be inefficient at moving the skeleton.

Cartilage, sometimes known as the "shock absorber" of the joint, is a strong, elastic tissue that surrounds the ends of bones. It creates a smooth surface for bones to slide across during movement, minimizing friction and protecting the bone surface. Furthermore, cartilage functions as a cushion, absorbing and spreading impact forces uniformly throughout the joint.

Injuries or degeneration of ligaments, tendons, or cartilage may have a major influence on joint function, causing discomfort, instability, and reduced mobility. Arthroscopic techniques address these concerns by mending or rebuilding damaged ligaments, removing damaged cartilage, or repairing torn tendons, therefore restoring joint stability and function.

How Joints Function

Joints serve as the meeting sites of bones, allowing for mobility and flexibility. The smooth surfaces of the bones inside a joint are coated with cartilage, allowing them to glide easily over one another during movement. Ligaments and tendons surround the joint and offer support while also allowing for regulated movement.

When a muscle contracts, it pulls on the tendon that connects to the bone, causing it to move. This movement takes place at the joint, where the bones contact. The range of motion is determined by the kind of joint used. For example, hinge joints, such as the knee, can only move in one direction (flexion and extension), but ball-and-socket joints, such as the hip, may move in numerous directions.

Muscles, tendons, ligaments, and cartilage work together to provide smooth, pain-free movement at the joints. However, if any component is injured or impaired, it may result in joint dysfunction, discomfort, and restricted motion.

Understanding joint function is critical for accurately identifying and treating joint diseases. Arthroscopic techniques use this expertise to examine and treat joint disorders, restoring function and alleviating discomfort.

Importance Of Joint Health

Joint health is essential for living an active, pain-free lifestyle. Healthy joints provide for smooth, painless mobility, enabling people to go about their everyday lives, exercise, and engage in sports and leisure activities without restrictions.

Regular exercise, adequate diet, weight control, and injury avoidance are all important aspects of maintaining joint health. Exercise strengthens the muscles around the joint, giving support and stability. It also improves flexibility and range of motion, which reduces the likelihood of injury and joint stiffness.

A nutritious diet high in calcium, vitamin D, and omega-3 fatty acids promotes bone and joint health. These nutrients serve to maintain cartilage integrity, increase bone density, and decrease inflammation, all of which contribute to overall joint function.

Maintaining a healthy weight is particularly important for joint health since excess weight may put additional stress on the joints, causing wear and tear and an increased risk of osteoarthritis. Individuals may protect their joints and lower their risk of future joint issues by living a healthy lifestyle that includes frequent exercise, a balanced diet, and weight control.

Understanding the significance of joint health enables people to make proactive efforts to maintain and preserve their joints, enabling them to live an active and pain-free lifestyle for many years. Arthroscopic operations are essential for maintaining joint health because they diagnose and treat joint issues early on, avoiding additional damage and preserving joint function.

CHAPTER 3

Preparing For Arthroscopic Surgery

Preoperative Exams And Testing

Patients often go through many pre-operative exams and tests before having arthroscopic surgery to ensure they are healthy enough for the treatment and to acquire information that will help the surgical team during the operation.

One of the most common exams is a physical examination performed by the surgeon. During this evaluation, the surgeon will assess the damaged joint for symptoms of inflammation, instability, or other complications that may influence the operation.

In addition to the physical examination, imaging studies may be requested to provide a better picture of the joint.

These tests may involve X-rays, MRI scans, or CT scans, depending on the patient's requirements and the suspected problem impacting the joint.

Blood tests are also often used to analyze the patient's general health and to look for any underlying medical issues that might impair the operation or healing process.

In rare circumstances, specialist testing may be requested depending on the patient's unique requirements and the suspected joint issue. These tests may involve ultrasound imaging, arthrography, or joint aspiration to collect a sample of synovial fluid for examination.

Overall, pre-operative exams and testing are critical to ensure that the surgical team has a thorough picture of the patient's health and the status of the afflicted joint before performing arthroscopic surgery.

Medications And Diet Restrictions

Patients are often urged to make changes to their medicines and diet before arthroscopic surgery to reduce the risk of problems during and after the treatment.

One typical recommendation is to temporarily halt the use of certain drugs that may increase the risk of bleeding after surgery. These treatments may include blood thinners like aspirin, warfarin, or nonsteroidal anti-inflammatory drugs (NSAIDs). Patients are often recommended to discontinue these drugs several days before surgery, with the direction of their healthcare physician.

In addition to modifying medicines, patients may be told to observe certain food restrictions in the days preceding surgery. This often entails fasting for a certain length of time before the treatment to ensure that the stomach is empty, lowering the chance of issues like aspiration during anesthesia.

Patients are often given precise instructions on which drugs to discontinue and when, as well as particular fasting protocols before surgery. To reduce the risk of problems and ensure the success of the arthroscopic treatment, patients should carefully follow these guidelines.

Arranging Transportation And Assistance

Another critical component of preparing for arthroscopic surgery is planning transportation to and from the operating facility, as well as assuring enough assistance during the recuperation time.

Patients are often not permitted to drive themselves home after having anesthesia, so they must arrange for transportation to and from the surgery center from a friend or family member. This guarantees that patients may securely return home following the treatment, without endangering themselves or others.

In addition to transportation, patients may need help with activities of daily life during the early stages of recuperation. This might involve assistance with domestic duties, food preparation, and personal care responsibilities like bathing and dressing.

Patients are urged to discuss their post-operative requirements with their healthcare practitioner and make any required preparations well in advance of the procedure. By ensuring that transportation and assistance are in place, patients may concentrate on their rehabilitation with confidence that their requirements will be met.

Mental Preparation For Surgery

Preparing psychologically for arthroscopic surgery is an essential part of the total preparation process because it may help patients deal with the stress and worry that comes with having surgery.

One technique for mental preparation is to learn about the process and what to anticipate before, during, and after surgery. This may assist in relieving anxieties and doubts by offering a more detailed explanation of what will occur at each step of the procedure.

Another effective option is to use relaxation techniques like deep breathing, meditation, or visualization to decrease anxiety and produce a feeling of peace and control. These strategies are particularly useful in the days leading up to surgery and just before entering the operating room.

Patients might also benefit from discussing any concerns or questions they have regarding the operation with their healthcare physician. Open and honest communication with the surgical team may help reduce worries and create trust, making the whole procedure seem more manageable.

In addition to these techniques, some patients find it beneficial to seek the emotional support of friends and family members during the pre-operative time. A robust support network may provide comfort and encouragement, making patients feel more secure and prepared for the upcoming operation.

CHAPTER 4

Arthroscopic Procedure

Overview Of The Surgical Process

Arthroscopy is a minimally invasive surgical treatment for diagnosing and treating joint disorders. It lets surgeons see, diagnose, and treat diseases within the joint using tiny incisions and a camera known as an arthroscope. This approach has various benefits over standard open surgery, including shorter recovery periods, less postoperative discomfort, and a lower chance of complications.

The surgical procedure starts with the patient being prepared for surgery, which includes cleaning the surgical site and giving an anesthetic. Once the patient is anesthetized, the surgeon makes tiny incisions around the joint to be checked or treated. These incisions are generally smaller than half an inch in length.

Anesthesia Options

Various anesthetic alternatives may be utilized during arthroscopic surgeries, depending on the circumstances and the patient and surgeon's preferences. Anesthesia may be administered locally, regionally, or generally.

Local anesthesia is the process of injecting drugs into the surgical region to numb it and provide pain relief during the treatment. Regional anesthesia numbs a wider part of the body, such as a complete limb, via nerve blocks or spinal anesthesia. General anesthesia causes a short loss of consciousness, enabling the patient to remain uninformed and painless during the procedure.

The intricacy of the treatment, the patient's general condition, and their preferences all influence the kind of anesthetic used. The anesthesia staff works closely with the surgeon to guarantee the patient's safety and comfort during the procedure.

Insertion Of Arthroscopes And Instruments

The surgeon puts the arthroscope into the joint via one of the tiny incisions once the anesthetic has taken effect. The arthroscope is a tiny, flexible tube fitted with a camera and light source that allows the surgeon to see the interior of the joint on a display.

Additional tiny incisions may be made to introduce specialized surgical equipment, such as probes, scissors, or shavers, for tissue manipulation and repair. These devices are specifically designed to fit through the tiny incisions formed during the process.

The surgeon gently guides the arthroscope and equipment through the joint, inspecting the structures and diagnosing any abnormalities or damage. The arthroscope's high-definition pictures allow for exact diagnosis and therapy of the underlying disease.

Visualizing And Treating Joints

With the arthroscope in place, the surgeon can see the whole joint, including the cartilage, ligaments, tendons, and synovium. Any damaged or diseased tissue may be discovered and treated during the operation.

Common arthroscopy procedures include mending torn ligaments or tendons, removing loose pieces of cartilage or bone, and smoothing damaged surfaces. In certain circumstances, more complex operations, such as cartilage grafting or joint repair, may be required.

Throughout the procedure, the surgeon evaluates the progress and makes adjustments to the treatment plan as required depending on the results. After any required repairs or interventions have been made, the devices are withdrawn and the wounds are closed with sutures or adhesive strips.

Following the surgery, the patient is transported to a recovery area and carefully observed while they awaken from anesthesia. Depending on the intricacy of the operation and individual conditions, patients may be able to go home the same day or need a brief hospital stay for monitoring. Rehabilitation and physical therapy are often prescribed to help with the healing process and improve the results after arthroscopic surgery.

CHAPTER 5

Recovery And Rehabilitation

Immediate Post-Operative Care

Following the arthroscopic operation, the immediate emphasis changes to post-operative care. This period is critical for a smooth recovery and reducing problems. Immediately after surgery, you will be brought to a recovery area where healthcare specialists will check your vital signs and assure your stability. Depending on the procedure's intricacy and your general health, you may be admitted to the hospital for a few hours or overnight for observation.

During this early period, it is usual to feel some soreness, swelling, and sometimes nausea or dizziness as a result of the anesthetic. Your medical staff will prescribe pain and nausea drugs as required. They will also check your incision sites for symptoms of bleeding or infection.

To help in the healing process, follow your surgeon's directions for wound care, medication regimen, and activity level. This may involve keeping the incision areas clean and dry, using prescription pain relievers as indicated, and refraining from activities that might strain the surgical region.

Pain Management Strategies

Effective pain management is critical for patient comfort and a speedy recovery after arthroscopy. Your surgeon will prescribe pain medication depending on your specific requirements and medical history. These might include over-the-counter pain medicines like acetaminophen or nonsteroidal anti-inflammatory drugs (NSAIDs), as well as harsher prescription treatments like opioids.

In addition to pharmaceuticals, several non-pharmacological pain management options may assist relieve discomfort throughout the healing process.

This may include:

• Ice packs may decrease swelling and numb surrounding tissues, offering pain relief after surgery.

• Elevating the injured limb above the heart helps decrease swelling, enhance circulation, and alleviate discomfort.

• Compression bandages or stockings may minimize swelling and offer support for the surgical region, thereby reducing discomfort.

If you're in continuous or severe pain, you should contact your medical team so that they can change your treatment plan appropriately.

Physical Therapy Exercises

Physical therapy is an important part of the post-arthroscopy recovery. Your surgeon may suggest that you begin physical therapy as soon as possible following the treatment to help restore strength, flexibility, and range of motion in the afflicted joint.

A qualified physical therapist will collaborate with you to create a personalized workout program based on your unique requirements and objectives.

These exercises might include:

• Gentle range-of-motion exercises may enhance joint flexibility and mobility.

• Strength training focuses on strengthening the muscles around the joint, providing stability and support.

• Balance and Proprioception Exercises: Enhance coordination and proprioception, lowering the risk of falls and injuries.

To get the greatest benefits, execute these exercises regularly and properly. Your physical therapist will walk you through each activity and track your progress to ensure that you are moving forward safely in your recovery.

Gradual Return To Normal Activities

As you go through the healing and rehabilitation process, your surgeon will advise you on when it is safe to gradually resume regular activities. This might involve going back to work, driving, and engaging in leisure or sporting activities.

It's critical to listen to your body and avoid pushing too hard, particularly in the first phases of recuperation. Gradually increase the intensity and length of activities as tolerated, paying close attention to any indicators of pain or discomfort. If you encounter any setbacks or persistent symptoms, contact your medical team for additional examination and advice.

By following your surgeon's instructions and actively engaging in the rehabilitation process, you may increase the success of your arthroscopy treatment and achieve a complete recovery.

CHAPTER 6

Complications And Risks

Potential Complications Of Arthroscopy

Arthroscopy, like any other medical treatment, has risks and possible problems. While it is usually regarded as safe, it is important to be aware of these risks.

Infection is one of the possible complications. Despite strict sterilizing processes in contemporary medical institutions, there is always a danger of infection when the skin is broken. Infection may cause redness, swelling, warmth, and increasing discomfort at the surgery site. In extreme situations, fever and chills may also develop. Prompt detection and treatment of infections is critical to avoiding additional problems.

Another potential risk is nerve or blood vessel injury. During arthroscopy, tools are introduced into the joint area, which increases the risk of injuring nearby nerves or blood vessels. This may cause numbness, tingling, weakness, and even loss of function in the afflicted limb. Careful maneuvering and exact skill by the surgeon assist in reducing this danger, but it remains a potential.

Furthermore, there is a danger of severe bleeding during or after the treatment. Although arthroscopy is minimally invasive, some bleeding is unavoidable. In rare situations, bleeding may become excessive, resulting in hematoma development or the need for a blood transfusion. Patients with bleeding problems or those using blood thinners are at greater risk and should notify their surgeon in advance.

Finally, problems from anesthesia may develop. While uncommon, adverse responses to anesthetic medicines or problems like respiratory depression may occur. Anesthesia physicians actively monitor patients during the treatment to reduce these risks, but patients must report any relevant medical history or concerns in advance.

Infection Prevention Measures

In arthroscopic surgery, infection prevention is the number one goal. Healthcare practitioners use a variety of methods to limit the risk of infection before, during, and after the surgery.

One critical step is appropriate skin preparation at the surgery site. This usually entails thorough cleansing with antiseptic solutions to lower the quantity of microorganisms on the skin's surface. To prevent germs from entering the surgical field, the surgical crew wears sterile gowns and gloves.

Furthermore, sterile drapes are employed to provide a barrier between the surgical site and the surrounding area. This helps to avoid contamination from airborne particles and contact with non-sterile surfaces.

Maintaining a sterile atmosphere during the surgery is critical to lowering the risk of infection.

Antibiotic prophylaxis is another significant method used to avoid infection. Patients may be given antibiotics before the treatment to help minimize the risk of surgical site infections. The kind of antibiotic used and the time of administration are determined by the patient's medical history, the type of treatment done, and local recommendations.

Proper handling and sanitation of surgical tools are also necessary for infection prevention. Before being used, instruments must be thoroughly cleaned and sterilized to guarantee that germs and other pollutants are removed. Regular maintenance of sterilizing equipment and adherence to prescribed standards reduce the incidence of instrument-related infections.

Finally, proper post-operative wound care is critical for infection prevention. Patients are given instructions on how to care for their surgical wounds, which include keeping the area clean and dry, changing dressings as required, and watching for symptoms of infection. Prompt reporting of any worrying symptoms to healthcare practitioners enables early detection and treatment if an infection develops.

Managing Postoperative Pain And Discomfort

It is typical to feel some pain and discomfort after arthroscopic surgery while the body recovers. However, there are several successful ways to treat postoperative pain.

Pain medicines are a popular treatment option. Patients with severe pain may be administered oral pain medications such as acetaminophen, nonsteroidal anti-inflammatory medicines (NSAIDs), or opioids. It is important to take these drugs as prescribed by the surgeon or healthcare practitioner and to be aware of any possible adverse effects or interactions with other medications.

In addition to oral drugs, local anesthetic procedures may be employed to numb the surgical site and give focused pain management. This may involve injecting local anesthetics or using nerve blocks to prevent pain signals from reaching the brain. These treatments may give instant comfort while perhaps reducing the need for systemic pain drugs.

Physical therapy and rehabilitation are also important aspects of pain treatment after arthroscopy. A planned exercise regimen may aid with range of motion, muscular strength, and joint healing. Physical therapists collaborate with patients to create unique treatment regimens based on their particular requirements and objectives.

Furthermore, cold treatment and elevation may help minimize swelling and discomfort after surgery. Ice packs may be applied to the surgical site for brief periods multiple times each day to help numb it and reduce inflammation. Elevating the afflicted leg above the level of the heart may help to remove extra fluid and minimize swelling.

Patients should talk honestly with their healthcare professionals about their pain levels and treatment choices. By collaborating, patients and physicians may create a comprehensive pain management plan that meets individual requirements and facilitates a smooth recovery.

Signs Of Complications To Watch For

While problems after arthroscopic surgery are uncommon, it is important to watch for any signs or symptoms that might signal a problem.

Infection is a typical issue to look for. Redness, swelling, warmth, and increasing discomfort at the surgery site are all signs of an infection. In certain circumstances, pus or discharge may be present. Additionally, fever and chills may suggest a systemic illness and should be reported to healthcare specialists right once.

Another possible risk is deep vein thrombosis (DVT), which happens when a blood clot develops in a deep vein, often in the leg. DVT symptoms include swelling, discomfort, tenderness, and redness in the afflicted leg. If left untreated, DVT may progress to more catastrophic consequences such as pulmonary embolism, which occurs when a blood clot moves to the lungs and stops blood flow.

Another worry after arthroscopic surgery is nerve or blood vessel injury. Nerve injury symptoms might include numbness, tingling, weakness, or lack of feeling in the afflicted limb. If blood vessels are injured, there may be excessive bleeding or the development of a hematoma.

Other possible consequences include allergic responses to drugs or anesthesia, anesthetic side effects, and surgical procedure-related issues such as insufficient healing or chronic discomfort.

Patients must carefully follow post-operative instructions and notify their healthcare professionals immediately if they have any odd symptoms or concerns. Early identification and management may assist in preventing issues from worsening and encourage a full recovery. Regular follow-up meetings with the surgeon or healthcare team are also necessary to monitor development and handle any concerns that may occur.

CHAPTER 7

Arthroscopy Of Specific Joints

Knee Arthroscopy: Procedures And Results

Knee arthroscopy is a minimally invasive surgical treatment that diagnoses and treats knee joint disorders. It entails putting a tiny camera called an arthroscope into the knee joint via small incisions. This lets the physician observe the interior of the knee on a monitor and execute any necessary surgical operations.

A typical cause for knee arthroscopy is to identify and repair meniscus tears. The meniscus is a rubbery C-shaped disk that cushions the knee joint. When it rips, it may cause discomfort, edema, and trouble moving the knee.

During knee arthroscopy, the surgeon may trim or repair the torn meniscus, depending on the degree of the tear.

Another typical problem treated during knee arthroscopy is the removal of loose bodies from the knee joint. These might be bone or cartilage pieces that have broken off, producing discomfort and limited mobility. Arthroscopy lets the surgeon find and remove loose bodies without making a big incision.

Knee arthroscopy may also be used to treat a variety of different diseases, including ligament tears (such as the anterior cruciate ligament, or ACL), cartilage damage, and synovitis. The particular technique used will be determined by the patient's condition and the surgeon's evaluation.

One of the primary advantages of knee arthroscopy is its minimum invasiveness. Compared to conventional open surgery, arthroscopy usually causes less discomfort, quicker recovery, and fewer scars. Patients may commonly go home the same day as their operation and return to regular activities within a few weeks.

However, it is important to remember that knee arthroscopy is not appropriate for all knee disorders. Some diseases may need more substantial surgery, such as a complete knee replacement. Patients should consult with their surgeon to identify the best course of action for their unique condition.

Knee arthroscopy is an effective technique for identifying and treating a variety of knee diseases. By enabling surgeons to view the joint and execute treatments with minimum invasiveness, patients may recover quicker and achieve better results.

Shoulder Arthroscopy: Indications And Benefits

Shoulder arthroscopy is a minimally invasive surgical treatment that diagnoses and treats shoulder joint disorders. It entails putting a tiny camera called an arthroscope into the shoulder joint via small incisions. This lets the physician see inside the shoulder on a monitor and execute different surgical operations as required.

One typical reason for shoulder arthroscopy is to repair damaged rotator cuff tendons. The rotator cuff is a collection of muscles and tendons that surround the shoulder joint and serve to support and move the arm. When these tendons rip, it may cause discomfort, weakness, and a restricted range of movement. Arthroscopic surgery enables the surgeon to access and mend damaged tendons using tiny devices and sutures.

Another typical condition treated during shoulder arthroscopy is shoulder joint instability. This might be related to ligament laxity or repetitive dislocations. During arthroscopic surgery, the surgeon may tighten and repair the ligaments around the shoulder joint, increasing stability and lowering the risk of future dislocations.

Shoulder arthroscopy may also be used to treat other problems such as labral tears (tears in the cartilage ring around the shoulder socket), impingement syndrome (compression of the rotator cuff tendons and bursa), and shoulder arthritis. The particular technique used will be determined by the patient's condition and the surgeon's evaluation.

One of the primary advantages of shoulder arthroscopy is its minimum invasiveness. Compared to conventional open surgery, arthroscopy usually causes less discomfort, quicker recovery, and fewer scars.

Patients may commonly go home the same day as their operation and return to regular activities within a few weeks.

However, it is important to highlight that shoulder arthroscopy is not appropriate for all shoulder conditions. Some diseases may need more substantial surgery, such as shoulder replacement. Patients should consult with their surgeon to identify the best course of action for their unique condition.

Shoulder arthroscopy is an effective technique for identifying and treating a variety of shoulder disorders. By enabling surgeons to view the joint and execute treatments with minimum invasiveness, patients may recover quicker and achieve better results.

Hip Arthroscopy: Applications And Limitations.

Hip arthroscopy is a minimally invasive surgical treatment that diagnoses and treats hip joint disorders.

It entails putting a tiny camera called an arthroscope into the hip joint via small incisions. This enables the physician to see inside the hip on a monitor and execute different surgical operations as required.

One typical reason for hip arthroscopy is to address femoroacetabular impingement (FAI). FAI occurs when the hip joint's bones come into improper contact, causing discomfort and limiting range of motion. During arthroscopic surgery, the surgeon might modify the bones of the hip joint to lessen friction and discomfort.

Another typical condition treated by hip arthroscopy is the correction of labral tears. The labrum is a cartilage ring that borders the rim of the hip socket and serves to keep the joint stable. Tears in the labrum may lead to hip discomfort, clicking, and instability. Arthroscopic surgery enables the physician to reach and repair the torn labrum using tiny tools and sutures.

Hip arthroscopy may also be performed to treat other disorders, including hip impingement, dysplasia, and synovitis. The particular technique used will be determined by the patient's condition and the surgeon's evaluation.

One of the limits of hip arthroscopy is its technical difficulty owing to the complicated anatomy of the hip joint. Not all hip disorders may be successfully addressed with arthroscopy, and some may need more comprehensive surgery, such as hip replacement. Patients should consult with their surgeon to identify the best course of action for their unique condition.

Hip arthroscopy is an effective technique for identifying and treating a variety of hip disorders. By enabling surgeons to view the joint and execute treatments with minimum invasiveness, patients may recover quicker and achieve better results.

Ankle And Wrist Arthroscopy: Special Considerations

Ankle and wrist arthroscopy are minimally invasive surgical techniques that detect and treat issues with the ankle and wrist joints, respectively. They, like other arthroscopic procedures, entail introducing a tiny camera known as an arthroscope into the joint via small incisions. This enables the physician to see inside the joint on a monitor and execute different surgical operations as required.

Ankle arthroscopy is often used to address ankle impingement, ankle instability, and cartilage injuries. The surgeon may employ arthroscopic methods to remove bone spurs, mend ligaments, and treat cartilage damage, among other things.

Wrist arthroscopy is often performed to diagnose and treat wrist arthritis, ligament tears (particularly scapholunate ligament tears), and ganglion cysts. The surgeon may employ arthroscopic methods to remove inflammatory tissue, mend ligaments, and remove cysts, among other things.

One benefit of ankle and wrist arthroscopy is that it is less invasive, resulting in less discomfort, quicker recovery, and smaller scars than standard open surgery. However, it is important to remember that not all ankle and wrist diseases may be successfully addressed with arthroscopy, and some may need more comprehensive surgery.

Finally, ankle and wrist arthroscopy are effective diagnostic and treatment methods for a variety of ankle and wrist issues. By enabling surgeons to view the joint and conduct minimally invasive operations, patients may benefit from speedier recovery and better results.

CHAPTER 8

Advanced Techniques And Innovation

Emerging Technology In Arthroscopic Surgery

Arthroscopic surgery, which was once a breakthrough leap in medical research, is still evolving as new technology emerges. These developments are intended to increase accuracy, reduce invasiveness, and improve patient outcomes. One important advancement is the incorporation of high-definition imaging equipment, which allows surgeons to see joint components more clearly throughout the process. This enables for more exact diagnosis and therapy.

Another growing technology is the creation of specialized devices and equipment, such as enhanced arthroscopes with smaller diameters and more agility. These instruments allow surgeons to more easily reach complicated parts of the joint, lowering the risk of tissue injury and increasing overall surgical efficiency.

Furthermore, the use of augmented reality (AR) and virtual reality (VR) devices has transformed preoperative planning and intraoperative navigation. Surgeons may now view the patient's anatomy in 3D, enabling more tailored and accurate treatment options. AR and VR also enable surgeons to get more comprehensive training by providing realistic simulations of surgical operations that help them improve their skills and expertise.

Minimally Invasive Approaches

One of the guiding concepts of arthroscopic surgery is its minimally invasive nature, which attempts to decrease stress on surrounding tissues and speed up the patient's recovery. Small incisions, usually less than one centimeter long, are used in minimally invasive procedures to introduce specialized equipment and cameras into the joint.

Minimally invasive procedures provide various benefits over standard open surgery, including less postoperative discomfort, shorter hospital stays, and a faster return to routine activities. These methods are very useful for treating diseases including meniscus tears, ligament injuries, and cartilage abnormalities.

In addition to smaller incisions, minimally invasive arthroscopic operations often include methods such as tissue-sparing approaches and selective tissue debridement, which preserve healthy tissue while addressing the particular disease. This reduces the risk of problems while also promoting speedier healing and recovery.

Future Trends In The Field

As technology advances, the future of arthroscopic surgery offers significant opportunities for additional innovation and advancement. One important trend is the development of artificial intelligence (AI) systems for predictive analytics and decision assistance during arthroscopy treatments. These AI-powered tools can analyze massive quantities of patient data to help surgeons plan treatments, forecast results, and improve surgical skills.

Furthermore, integrating new materials and biologics into arthroscopic treatments has the potential to transform tissue healing and regeneration. Biomaterial scaffolds, growth factors, and stem cell treatments provide promising potential for improving tissue repair and long-term joint health.

Furthermore, the ongoing advancement of minimally invasive methods and equipment will allow surgeons to execute increasingly difficult surgeries with better accuracy and speed. This includes innovations in endoscopic methods, such as single-port arthroscopy and wireless instrumentation, which reduce surgical trauma and increase patient satisfaction.

The area of arthroscopic surgery is constantly developing with the introduction of new technology, less invasive techniques, robotic help, and future developments. These developments not only improve surgical results but also overall patient care and quality of life. As technology advances, the opportunities for innovation and improvement in arthroscopic surgery expand, providing a better future for both patients and surgeons.

CHAPTER 9

Lifestyles And Prevention

Maintaining Joint Health With Exercise And Diet

Exercise and nutrition are critical in maintaining joint health and functioning. Regular physical exercise promotes joint flexibility, strength, and general mobility. Exercises that target particular muscle groups around the joints may assist in reducing tension and strain on the joints.

Low-impact workouts, such as swimming, cycling, and walking, are ideal alternatives for supporting joint health since they reduce joint strain while delivering a cardiovascular workout. Furthermore, strength training activities that target the muscles that support the joints, such as squats and lunges, may assist to stabilize and protect them.

A well-balanced diet high in nutrients is also necessary for joint health. Fish, flaxseeds, and walnuts contain omega-3 fatty acids, which have anti-inflammatory qualities and may help to alleviate joint pain and stiffness caused by disorders such as arthritis. Similarly, meals strong in antioxidants, such as fruits and vegetables, may assist in reducing inflammation and oxidative stress, hence improving joint health.

Hydration is another important part of joint health. Drinking enough water throughout the day helps to keep your joints lubricated, minimizing friction and avoiding pain when moving. Incorporating these lifestyle behaviors into your daily routine will greatly help to maintain joint health and general well-being.

Injury Prevention Strategies

Preventing injuries is critical for preserving joint health and general physical function. Understanding the most frequent causes of joint injuries, such as rapid hits, repeated motions, and overuse, may help people take proactive steps to reduce their risk.

Proper warm-up and stretching procedures before physical activity may assist in preparing the muscles and joints for movement, lowering the risk of strains and sprains. Wearing suitable protective gear, such as supportive footwear and joint braces, may also give additional protection during high-risk tasks.

Maintaining proper posture and body mechanics is critical for injury prevention, particularly while doing repeated actions or heavy lifting. Proper lifting methods and avoiding quick, jerky motions may assist in reducing stress on the joints and surrounding tissues.

Regular rest and recovery intervals are also important for avoiding overuse injuries. Allowing the body enough time to recuperate between exercises promotes tissue repair and regeneration, lowering the likelihood of chronic joint disorders.

Ergonomics And Joint-Friendly Habits

Ergonomics is the design of workplaces and equipment to improve human performance while lowering the risk of damage. Implementing ergonomic concepts in the office and at home may improve joint health and general comfort.

Maintaining optimal workplace ergonomics, such as altering chair height and monitoring position to achieve neutral joint alignment, may aid in the prevention of musculoskeletal disorders including back and neck discomfort. Similarly, employing ergonomic tools and equipment, such as keyboards and mouse pads, may help to lessen wrist and hand strain when using a computer.

Including joint-friendly practices in your everyday routine may also assist in lowering the chance of strain and injury. This includes avoiding lengthy periods of sitting or standing in the same posture, taking frequent pauses to stretch and move about, and carrying heavy things with good body mechanics.

The Need For Regular Check-Ups And Screenings

Regular check-ups and screenings are critical for discovering any joint problems early on and taking proper action to avoid additional harm. Routine physical exams by a healthcare expert may help detect indicators of joint dysfunction or underlying disorders that may need treatment.

Screenings such as bone density tests and imaging investigations may give important information about the health of the joints and surrounding tissues. Early identification of disorders like osteoporosis or arthritis enables early intervention techniques to be applied, perhaps averting future loss of joint function.

In addition to physical tests and screenings, open communication with healthcare practitioners is critical for treating any joint-related concerns or symptoms. Seeking immediate medical assistance for acute injuries or chronic joint pain may help to avoid long-term problems and ensure the best possible results. Regular check-ups and screenings are proactive methods for maintaining joint health and quality of life.

CHAPTER 10

After Surgery: Long-Term Joint Care

Follow-Up Appointments, Monitoring

Following an arthroscopy, follow-up consultations are critical to ensure that your joint recovers correctly and you regain full function. These consultations are usually planned within a few weeks after the operation, enabling your doctor to evaluate your progress, discuss any concerns, and make any required changes to your treatment plan.

During these follow-up appointments, your doctor will inspect the surgery site, measure your range of motion, and check for any residual symptoms like pain or edema. They may also prescribe imaging tests, such as X-rays or MRI scans, to obtain a better look at the joint and verify it is healing properly.

It is critical to attend all planned follow-up visits and discuss honestly with your healthcare provider about any changes or concerns you have observed following your surgery. By being proactive and involved in your rehabilitation, you can help assure the greatest possible result for your joint health.

Managing Chronic Conditions

While arthroscopy may help with specific joint disorders, it is important to note that surgery may not treat underlying chronic illnesses like osteoarthritis or rheumatoid arthritis. Managing these diseases requires a multifaceted strategy that may involve medication, physical therapy, lifestyle changes, and regular monitoring.

Your healthcare professional will collaborate with you to create a customized treatment plan that is suited to your requirements and objectives. This may include pain and inflammatory drugs, as well as methods for joint protection and long-term function.

In addition to medicinal treatments, self-care techniques such as regular exercise, keeping a healthy weight, and preserving your joints from overuse may all help you manage chronic joint disorders. By actively participating in your treatment and making educated decisions, you may help reduce symptoms and enhance your overall quality of life.

Coping With Limitations And Adaptive Activities

Following arthroscopy, you may have temporary limits in your ability to do particular tasks or engage in sports and leisure activities. Listen to your body and don't push yourself too hard throughout the recuperation process.

Your healthcare physician or physical therapist might recommend safe activities and exercises to help regain strength and flexibility in the damaged joint. They may also suggest changes or alternate approaches to activities that might aggravate symptoms or impede recovery.

In certain circumstances, you may need to make more major changes to your lifestyle or daily activities to accommodate persistent joint problems. This might include utilizing assistive equipment like braces or orthotics, changing your home or work environment to lessen joint stress, or looking into alternate types of exercise or enjoyment that are easier on your body.

Resources And Support For Maintaining Joint Health

Maintaining good joint health is a lifetime commitment that needs consistent work and assistance. Fortunately, there are several tools available to assist you along the process, including healthcare experts, support groups, and instructional publications.

Your healthcare practitioner may refer you to services such as physical therapists, dietitians, and pain management experts who can provide further advice and assistance targeted to your specific requirements. Support groups and online forums may also be helpful sources of encouragement and knowledge, enabling you to connect with others who are dealing with similar issues.

Educating oneself about your disease and treatment alternatives is another critical component of maintaining good joint health. Staying educated and proactive will allow you to make empowered choices about your treatment and successfully advocate for your needs.

By using these tools and actively engaging in your treatment, you may improve your joint health and have a meaningful and active lifestyle for many years to come.

Conclusion

Finally, arthroscopy represents a significant achievement in the area of orthopedic surgery, changing the detection and treatment of joint-related problems. In this detailed guide, we dived into the complexities of arthroscopy operations, giving light on their development, methods, uses, and advantages.

Arthroscopy has arisen as a less invasive procedure with significant benefits over standard open surgery. Its capacity to give good sight of the joint interior, along with minimum tissue damage, leads to decreased discomfort, quicker recovery periods, and a lower risk of problems for patients. Furthermore, smaller incisions provide better cosmetic results, increasing patient satisfaction.

One of the main advantages of arthroscopy is its adaptability. It applies to a variety of joints, including the knee, shoulder, hip, ankle, elbow, and wrist, enabling surgeons to treat a broad range of disorders such as ligament tears, cartilage damage, joint inflammation, and loose bodies. The introduction of specialized equipment and imaging methods has broadened the scope of arthroscopy treatments, allowing surgeons to treat complicated diseases with greater accuracy and effectiveness.

Furthermore, advances in arthroscopy technology continue to improve its capabilities. High-definition cameras, enhanced lighting systems, and specialized equipment all help to increase joint visualization and manipulation capabilities. The combination of robots and augmented reality has great potential for improving surgical precision and outcomes, paving the way for the future of arthroscopic surgery.

The advantages of arthroscopy go beyond the operating room. Its minimally invasive nature results in economic savings for healthcare systems, since shorter hospital stays and fewer rehabilitation needs lower total healthcare costs.

Furthermore, the ability to conduct numerous treatments as an outpatient improves patient convenience and access to care.

However, despite its tremendous benefits, arthroscopy has limits. Certain problems may still need open surgical surgery for best results, and patient selection is critical in assessing the suitability of arthroscopic therapy. Furthermore, continued research is required to develop procedures, broaden indications, and improve patient outcomes.

Finally, arthroscopy has transformed the care of joint problems by providing patients with a less intrusive and more effective method of diagnosis and treatment. As technology and surgical skills progress, the future offers promise for arthroscopy's role in improving musculoskeletal health and quality of life.

THE END

www.ingramcontent.com/pod-product-compliance
Lightning Source LLC
Chambersburg PA
CBHW071839210526
45479CB00001B/207